CW01375876

Mediterranean Diet Low Cholesterol Cookbook

Fast and Easy Low Cholesterol
Recipes to Make Healthy
Eating Delicious Every Day

By Nancy Marchetti

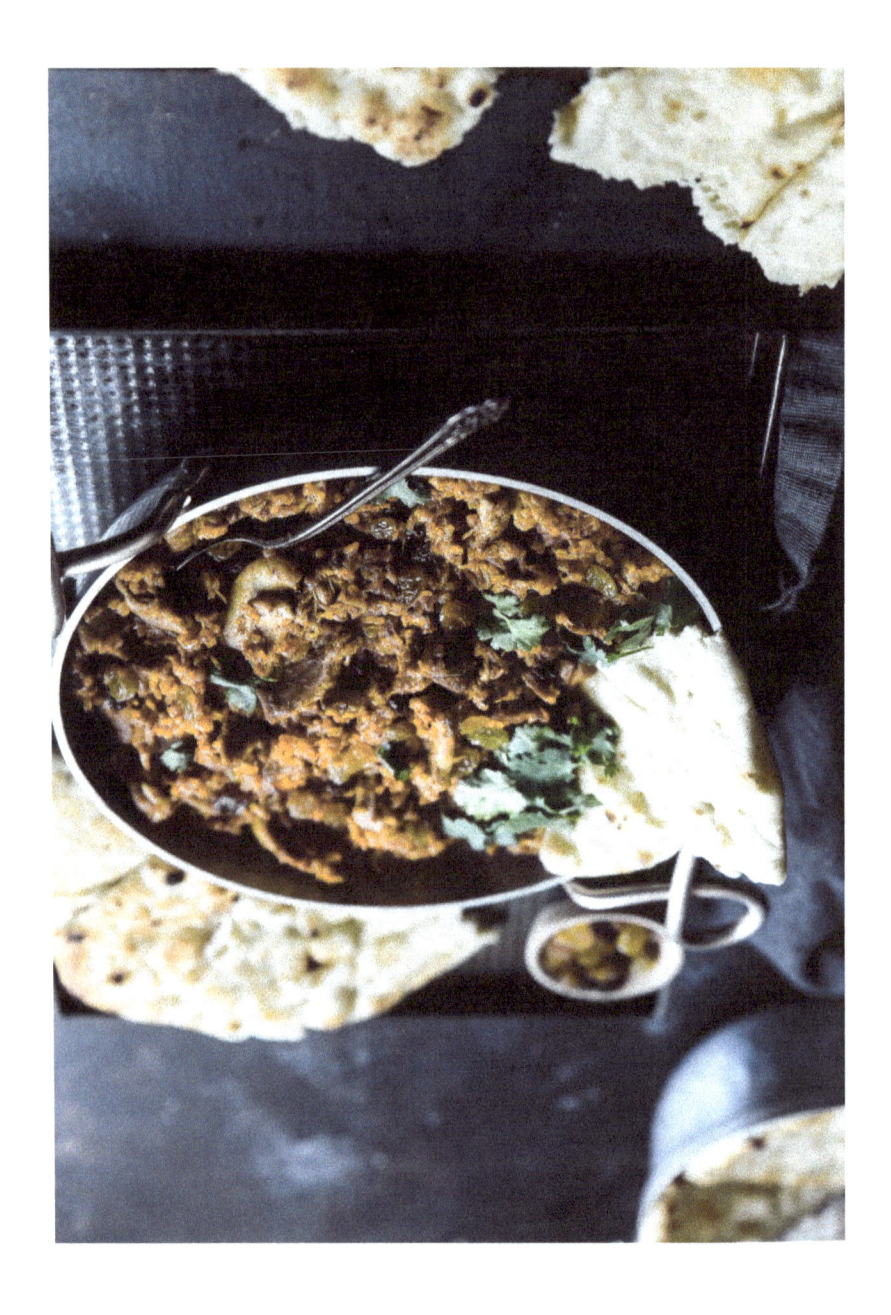

Copyright © Nancy Marchetti All rights reserved.

No part of this guide may be reproduced in any form without permission in writing from the publisher except in the case of brief quotations embodied in critical articles or reviews.

Legal & Disclaimer

The information contained in this book and its contents is not designed to replace or take the place of any form of medical or professional advice; and is not meant to replace the need for independent medical, financial, legal or other professional advice or services, as may be required. The content and information in this book has been provided for educational and entertainment purposes only.

The content and information contained in this book has been compiled from sources deemed reliable, and it is accurate to the best of the Author's knowledge, information and belief. However, the Author cannot guarantee its accuracy and validity and cannot be held liable for any errors and/or omissions. Further, changes are periodically made to this book as and when needed. Where appropriate and/or necessary, you must consult a professional (including but not limited to your doctor, attorney, financial advisor or such other professional advisor) before using any of the suggested remedies, techniques, or information in this book.

Upon using the contents and information contained in this book, you agree to hold harmless the Author from and against any damages, costs, and expenses, including any legal fees potentially resulting from the application of any of the information provided by this book. This disclaimer applies to any loss, damages or injury caused by the use and application, whether directly or indirectly, of any advice or information presented, whether for breach of contract, tort, negligence, personal injury, criminal intent, or under any other cause of action.

You agree to accept all risks of using the information presented inside this book.

You agree that by continuing to read this book, where appropriate and/or necessary, you shall consult a professional (including but not limited to your doctor, attorney, or financial advisor or such other advisor as needed) before using any of the suggested remedies, techniques, or information in this book.

Table of Contents

INTRODUCTION TO MEDITERRANEAN DIET 9

LOW CHOLESTEROL RECIPES 15

Mediterranean salad..15

Mediterranean salad with pasta...16

Mediterranean salad with tricolor pasta 18

Mediterranean chicken sitting..20

Mediterranean fish fillet..22

Mediterranean-inspired chickpea salad 24

Mediterranean spaghetti...26

Spaghetti Mediterráneo 27

Mediterranean-style baked fish 28

Mediterranean chayote..30

Mediterranean pizza...32

Mediterranean Frittata 35

Mediterranean shrimp..37

Greek or Mediterranean Sandwich 39

Mediterranean salad..41

Mediterranean pasta..42

Mediterranean salad spinach...44

Mediterranean style Fusilli salad 46

Roast vegetables and Arabic bread 47

Shrimp enchiladas 48

Mediterranean salad..50

Chickpea salad - Mediterranean...51

Mediterranean rolls 52

Mediterranean beef casserole 54

Mediterranean tuna salad 56

Mediterranean Screws 57

Mediterranean chicken with 4 cheeses 58

Grape salad 59

Slow Baked Beef 60

Baked Chicken in its Juice..62

Beef Meatballs in Vegetable Bath 63

Rice with Smoked Sausages and Beer 66

Red beef tail 68

Oven fried chicken thigh 70

Moro Red Beans with Salami Genoa 72

Dominican style coconut fish 74

MEDITERRANEAN SALAD 76
MEDITERRANEAN FISH CASSEROLE 77
MEDITERRANEAN SPOONS............... 79
MEDITERRANEAN SALAD IN LOW CHOLESTEROL 80
MEDITERRANEAN ORZO PASTA SALAD............... 83
MEDITERRANEAN TOAST WITH SEEDS 85
MAIN COURSE MEDITERRANEAN SALAD............... 86
MEDITERRANEAN SALAD WITH CHEESE 88
MEDITERRANEAN PASTA TOMATOES 89
MURCIAN MEDITERRANEAN PIZZA 90
MEDITERRANEAN CHICKPEA AND PASTA SALAD............... 92
BAKED MEDITERRANEAN SKIMMED 94
MEDITERRANEAN ROAST CHICKEN CHICKPEA SALAD............... 96
MEDITERRANEAN SALAD WITH TOMATOES............... 98
MEDITERRANEAN BRUSCHETTA............... 99

CONCLUSION 101

INTRODUCTION TO MEDITERRANEAN DIET

The Mediterranean recipes diet has been tailored from the foods and recipes found within the sixteen countries bordering the sea. several nowadays consider Mediterranean food because the same as Greek food. though Greek food is extremely a lot of a similar, the opposite bordering countries have had an outsized influence. change of state strategies grew out of a rural manner wherever the vegetables, herbs, and alternative ingredients area unit domestically adult by tiny farmers. several herbs and greens that area unit adult within the wild are used. Olive and lemon trees that area unit 2 necessary elements of Mediterranean change of state, grow well within the region. Locals use several herbs and spices like garlic, oregano, mint, thyme, and basil in their preparation. Foods area unit unbroken as contemporary as attainable, and people that area unit au gratin area unit au gratin terribly slowly with the freshest of ingredients giving flavors time to meld. Red meat is typically ingested no quite once a month. as a result of the population is therefore about to the ocean, fish may be a mainstay within the diet. Fish, in conjunction with organically created cheeses, oils, fruits, nuts, grains, legumes, and vegetables, area unit the idea of their diet. Water in giant quantities is additionally consumed often, and vino is consumed carefully. Sweets area unit typically consumed in fruits that area unit lower in calories and far higher in fiber and nutrients than sugared pastries. Because of the high use of vegetables and legumes and virtually no saturated fat, cardiovascular disease is found a lot of less usually than within the USA or alternative countries whose diets area unit high in red meats and dairy farm. The the big apple Times and U.S. News and World Report reported on initial studies indicating a attainable reduction in Alzheimer's disease in folks following this kind of diet. The Mediterranean recipes diet has been tailored from the foods and recipes found within the sixteen countries bordering the sea. several nowadays consider Mediterranean food because the same as Greek food. though Greek food is extremely a lot of a similar, the opposite bordering countries have had an outsized influence. change of state strategies grew out of a rural manner wherever the vegetables, herbs, and alternative ingredients area unit domestically adult by tiny farmers. several herbs and greens that area unit adult within the wild are used. Olive and lemon trees that area unit 2 necessary elements of Mediterranean change of state, grow well within the region. Locals use several herbs and spices like garlic, oregano, mint, thyme, and basil in their preparation. Foods area unit unbroken as contemporary as attainable, and people that area unit au gratin area unit au gratin terribly slowly with the freshest of ingredients giving flavors time to meld. Red meat is typically ingested no quite once a month. as a result of the population is therefore about to the ocean, fish may be a mainstay within the diet. Fish and organically created cheeses, oils, fruits, nuts, grains, legumes, and vegetables area unit the idea of their diet. Water in giant quantities is additionally consumed often, and vino is consumed carefully. Sweets area unit typically consumed in fruits that area unit lower in calories and far higher in fiber and nutrients than sugared pastries. Because of the high use of vegetables and legumes and virtually no saturated fat, cardiovascular disease is found a lot of less usually than within the USA or alternative countries whose diets area unit high in red meats and dairy farm. The the big apple Times and U.S. News and World Report reported on initial studies indicating a attainable reduction in Alzheimer's disease in folks following this kind of diet. In the last ten years, fashionable science has been investigation and proving the various helpful effects of the Mediterranean diet. It has, of course, been the staple diet of southern Europeans for many years, however because of airplanes, we are able to all eat this fashion. Here area unit four smart reasons to provide it a strive. You will slenderize Eating healthy food au gratin with a touch of care and smart fats is verified to assist you slenderize. you do not ought to eat the maximum amount to feel full, and what you are doing eat is full of vitamins and minerals. exploitation any of the various Mediterranean instruction books can see you losing the maximum amount as ten pounds a month painlessly. You will facilitate your heart The Mediterranean diet involves ingestion many contemporary fruit and vegetables, oily fish, and vegetable oil as a dressing. Oily fish and vegetable oil area unit wealthy sources of necessary mono and unsaturated fats. These fats area unit smart for you, creating your blood less sticky, lowering your sterol, and maintaining you in nice condition. the possibilities of obtaining cardiovascular disease area unit a lot of reduced. Less likelihood of cancer Being overweight may be a verified risk issue for several kinds of cancer. ingestion a Mediterranean-type diet not solely reduces your weight, however an outsized variety of vitamins and minerals facilitate to fight the free radicals your cells turn out daily. Beat cardiovascular disease If usually known as the silent killer, high pressure level shows no signs of it till you've got a coronary failure or a stroke. High pressure level is closely associated with being overweight and a poor diet. By following the Mediterranean diet, not solely does one slenderize, however you furthermore may eat less salt, each of that lower your pressure level. several studies have shown low levels of vitamins and minerals in many of us with cardiovascular disease. several vitamins and minerals you eat daily with the Mediterranean diet correct this to nice result. The Mediterranean diet helps alternative conditions like polygenic disease, metabolic syndrome, and constipation. it is easy to follow, and most recipes area unit fast and nutritive. provides it a go, and you may shortly feel nice. Due to its nice form of contemporary and colourful ingredients, the Mediterranean diet has become, for many, one in every of the tastiest and healthiest diets. UNESCO has recognized it as Intangible Cultural Heritage of Humanity for its stress on cordial reception, intercultural dialogue, and ability. By following a Mediterranean diet, complicated flavors area unit discovered, plentiful amounts of healthy fats area unit consumed, like people who return from vegetable oil and fatty fish (sardines, anchovies, mackerel, etc.), and wealthy sources of proteins area unit ready like meat and eggs. This diet additionally includes contemporary vegetables like bell peppers, aubergines, and zucchini, wealthy in plant product and facilitate keep you full for extended. We hope that this assortment of Mediterranean recipes helps you eat healthier and causes you to fancy and share your meals along with your family and friends within the purest Mediterranean vogue. as a result of as they are saying in European nation, "the best medication is nice change of state." Benefits of the Mediterranean diet for health Research shows that the Mediterranean diet has broad health edges, together with reducing liver fat volume or reducing symptoms related to depression. The Mediterranean diet combined with an occasional macromolecule diet will be particularly helpful for folks with polygenic disease. In this assortment, you may realize concepts for breakfasts, meals, snacks, and desserts which will assist you expertise the virtues of a Mediterranean diet low in carbohydrates or keto and pleasantly.

LOW CHOLESTEROL RECIPES

Mediterranean salad

Time: 30 minutes

Servings: 2

Ingredients

- 1/2 cubed cucumber
- 5 sliced radishes
- 1 lemon, its juice
- to taste shall
- to taste Pepper
- to taste mix of green leaves
- 1/2 cup filleted mushrooms
- 1/2 cup Bell pepper

Steps:

1) Wash and disinfect the green leaves, mushrooms and radishes. Mix all ingredients

Mediterranean salad with pasta

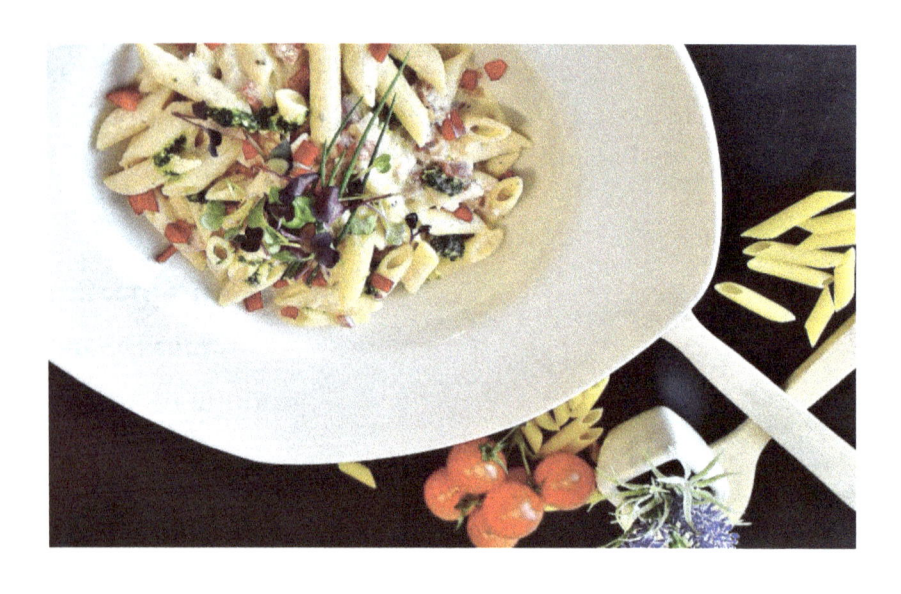

Time: 30 minutes

Servings: 6

Ingredients

- 400 gr penne pasta
- ¾ mug black pitted olives in half
- 6 cherry tomatoes halved
- 1/3 cup capers
- 1 aubergine girl
- 1 Red pepper
- 2 cdas olive oil
- 1 tooth it
- ¼ cup White vinegar

- ½ cup olive oil
- 1/3 cup chopped parsley
- Salt and pepper

Steps:

1) Cook the pasta and reserve.
2) Crush the garlic with half the vinegar, salt and half the oil. Reserve.
3) In a pan, put the two tablespoons of oil, pass the pepper and tomatoes.
4) Sauté the aubergines with salt and pepper.
5) Add the pasta with the olives, capers, and the dressing from steps 2, 3, and 4. Garnish with parsley.

Mediterranean salad with tricolor pasta

Time: 30 minutes

Servings: 6

Ingredients

- 400 gr mezze penne tricolor pasta
- ¾ mug black pitted olives in half
- 6 cherry tomatoes cut in half
- 1/3 cup small capers
- 1 small girl white eggplant
- 1 chopped red bell pepper
- 2 cdas olive oil
- 1 tooth it
- ¼ cup White vinegar
- ½ cup olive oil
- 1/3 cup chopped parsley
- Salt and pepper

Steps:

1) We put the salted water on the fire, when it breaks the boil, add the pasta according to the manufacturer's instructions and reserve.
2) In a mortar, crush the garlic with half the vinegar, salt and half the oil. Reserve.

3) Sauté the pepper and tomatoes in a pan with 2 tablespoons of oil, add the aubergines, salt and pepper to taste.

4) Mix the pasta with the olives, capers and garlic dressing. Add the peppers, tomatoes and aubergines.

5) Serve and garnish with the parsley.

Mediterranean chicken sitting

Time: 30 minutes

Servings: 4

Ingredients

- 1 whole chicken
- c/n vinaigrette
- c/n dads chambray
- c/n Cambray onion
- c/n carrots
- to taste chili that you like
- c/n wASHED OUT
- c/n romero
- to taste Wild salt from the natural sea
- 1 years beer

Steps:

1) Moisten the chicken with the vinaigrette 24 hours before and refrigerate it, add the rosemary and salt
2) Preheat the oven 15 min to 250 degrees 15 minutes
3) Preheat the oven 15 min to 250 degrees 15 minutes
4) Sit the chicken and put it in the oven
5) Mix the vegetables with the leftover vinaigrette from the chicken bowl
6) Cover the hole with a potato

7) Put the legumes together with the chicken

8) Put the chicken in the oven at 180 degrees

Mediterranean fish fillet

Time: 30 minutes

Servings: 2

Ingredients

- 2 steaks fish (Huauchinango, Robalo, Pargo, sea bream, etc.)
- 1-2 tomatoes
- 1 years tomato puree
- black olives needed
- 1-2 teeth it
- parsley
- shall
- Pepper
- 1 papa
- olive oil

Steps:

1) In a saucepan we put olive oil and a clove of minced garlic to brown when it releases the aroma we add one or two peeled and chopped tomatoes, then we add tomato puree, season with salt and pepper and add a potato peeled and cut into cubes of 1 cm., add some olives and chopped parsley.

2) When the potatoes have been cooked, carefully place the fish fillets to cook over low heat, if necessary add a little water.

3) Serve them with white rice.

Mediterranean-inspired chickpea salad

Time: 10 minutes + 1 hour rest

Servings: 2

Ingredients

- 1 years chickpeas, drained and rinsed
- 1 cup colored tomatoes in halves
- 1/2 small cucumber, peeled and cut in Macedonian
- 1 small red bell pepper cut into fruit salad
- 2 cdas capers
- 10 kalamata olives, halved lengthwise
- 1 slice onion (about 5 cm) cut into a feather
- 1 cdita oregano
- 1 good jet of sherry vinegar
- 1 board of directors organic EV olive oil
- 1 fist parsley cut into chifonada
- 3 black pepper mill turns
- Leaves French lettuce for serving (optional)

Steps:

1) Put all the ingredients except the parsley and lettuce in a bowl.
2) Mix and refrigerate for at least an hour
3) Mix occasionally so that the flavors blend well

4) Add the parsley just before serving. (So that it does not wilt) mix and serve on lettuce leaves or in a bowl.

Mediterranean spaghetti

Time: 30 minutes

Servings: 2

Ingredients

- 500 gr spaghetti
- 1 years black olives
- 2 ball tomatoes
- 3 cdas Extra virgin olive oil
- 3 twigs fresh basil
- 1 onion
- to taste shall
- to taste Pepper

Steps

1) In a pot you put water to boil and add the onion, halved with a little salt
2) Once it boils, you open your spaghetti and put it in the pot for about 20 minutes. Since your pasta is al dente, strain it removing the remains of the onion and take it to your refractory
3) In a frying pan you put the olive oil, as hot you add your chopped tomato and then the olives and serve it on your spaghetti, garnish with the basil leaves and you are ready to enjoy it.

Spaghetti Mediterráneo

Time: 25 minutes

Servings: 2

Ingredients

- 125 grs # 5 spaghetti
- 4 cdas olive oil
- 4 teeth it
- 2 branches parsley
- 1 tomato
- 4 olives
- 1 pinch basil
- 1/2 tsp bouillon powder

Steps

1) To make it, we cook the spaghetti in salted water. In a saucepan we put olive oil, 4 minced garlic cloves, a little chopped parsley, about 4 sliced olives and a peeled tomato, removed the seeds and cut into squares and season with half a teaspoon of powdered bouillon. When the al dente spaghetti is cooked, we light the oil with everything and when the garlic begins to smell we add the spaghetti and season with a pinch of basil.

Mediterranean-style baked fish

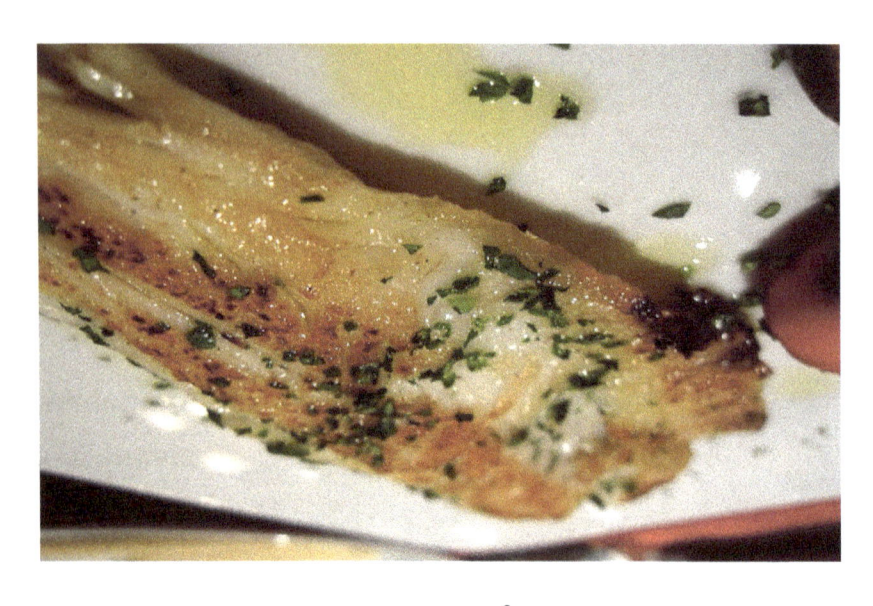

Time: 20 minutes

Servings: 2

Ingredients

- 1 steak fish per person
- 3 cebollitas de cambray
- 1 tooth garlic for each fillet
- red onion or échalots
- shall
- Pepper
- dill powder
- olive oil
- Butter

- capers (optional)
- 2 lemons

Steps

1) In a refractory we place our fish fillets on a little olive oil, and we are putting on top: each one: salt and pepper, a clove of minced garlic, minced red onion or échalots, the tails of about 3 small onions Chopped chambray and the onions are cut in half and placed on the sides, dill powder, a few capers, the juice of a lemon, olive oil and on top a piece of butter each.

2) It is put in a hot oven and you have to be on the lookout because it should not be more than 8 or 10 minutes so that it does not dry out. When we remove it, we decorate the fillets with lemon slices.

3) It's excellent.

Mediterranean chayote.

Time: 40 minutes

Servings: 6

Ingredients

- 1 kilogram tender chayotes
- 4 tablespoons olive oil
- 3 chives cut into rings, we are also going to use the stalks
- 3 teeth very minced garlic
- 3/4 kg tomatoes, peeled, seeded and finely chopped
- 1 tablespoon minced parsley
- 1 tablespoon minced thyme

Steps

1) The first thing we will do is peel the chayotes and cook them from cold salted water, or you can use a steamer.

2) Cut the two ends and cut them into very thin slices, in width or length, you decide.

3) In a frying pan, heat the oil, so that the onion and garlic are shredded, so they do not brown. Add the chopped tomatoes, cook over high heat to thicken the sauce, season with salt and pepper, sprinkle with the parsley.

4) Once the chayotes are cooked, drain them very well and dollars in the remaining oil, remove the excess fat with absorbent paper.

5) Bathe the chayotes with the tomato sauce, and sprinkle with the thyme to garnish.

6) Bon Appetite.

Mediterranean pizza

Time: 40 minutes

Servings: 6

Ingredients

For pizza

- 1/2 Pepper cut into strips
- 2 cdas pitted green olives, chopped
- 2 cdas pitted black olives, chopped
- 2 cdas Arugula finely chopped
- 2 tomatoes cut into thin slices
- 1 board of directors fresh basil
- 1 cdita Dried oregano
- 1 board of directors olive oil
- 100 gr Grated mozzarella cheese
- to taste Parmesan
- to taste Pepper
- to taste Salami (optional)
- For the sauce
- 1 cdta accept olive or canola
- 1 cdta shall
- 1 pinch sugar
- to taste Oregano (I recommend what fits in the palm of your hand)

- to taste Ground black pepper
- 2 teeth finely chopped garlic (can be garlic powder)
- 4 Fresh tomatoes
- 1/2 cup tomato puree
- 1/4 cup Water

For the mass
- 400 grams wheat flour
- 200 ml warm water
- 2 tablespoons olive oil
- 15 grams fresh yeast
- 1 pinch shall
- to taste Fine herbs
- c/n Flour for the surface (so it doesn't stick)

Steps

1) In a bowl we add the oil, water and yeast. Mix and then add the flour and a pinch of salt. Once we have more or less mixed everything in the bowl, we pass it to a surface, to knead well.

2) Now the kneading begins. We put a little flour on the surface and we will have to knead like 3 or 4 minutes without stopping. We will see that we have finished when the dough is completely smooth, if it sticks a lot we add a little flour and continue until it is smooth.

3) Once ready, we let it rest for 1 hour or so. Once settled, we split it in two and we can make two pizzas. We knead and stretch it.

4) To prepare the sauce, brown the garlic in the oil over low heat, add the oregano, salt, sugar, pepper and add the blended tomato and tomato puree, stir slowly until all the ingredients are incorporated Without stopping stirring, add the water, continue stirring until it boils for the first time, remove from heat and blend. This sauce can be used in pizza, Spaghetti Bolognese or other dishes based on this sauce.

5) Spread the sauce on all the pizza, evenly, then sprinkle the mozzarella cheese, finally add all the vegetables and salami at our discretion.

6) Season with the olive oil, salt and pepper.

7) We sprinkle a little fresh oregano and Parmesan cheese.

Mediterranean Frittata

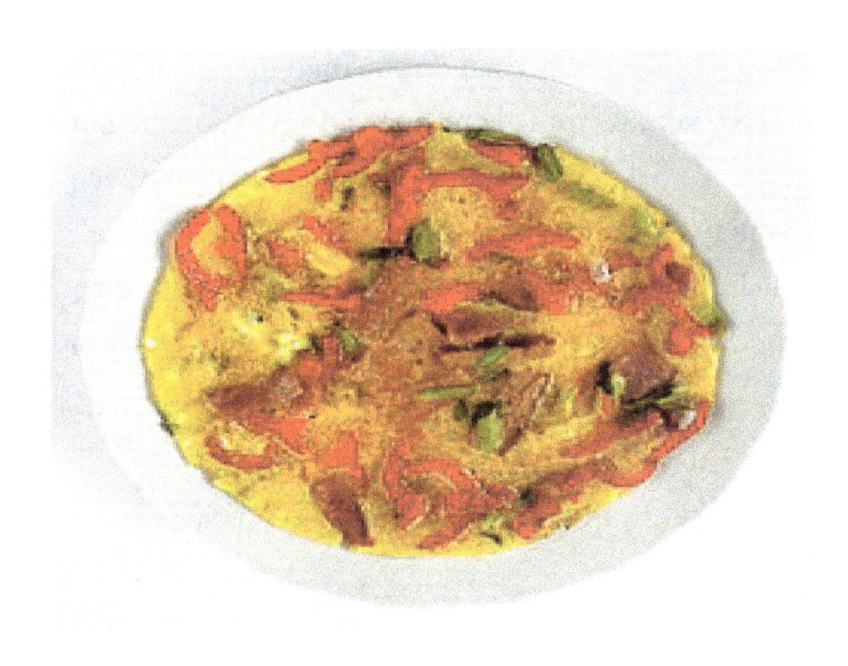

Time: 30 minutes

Servings: 4

Ingredients

- 3 eggs
- 1 splash milk
- to taste Pepper
- 2 mushrooms
- 1 piece purple Onion
- 1 fist olives
- 1 fist capers
- 1/2 Red pepper

- 1/2 yellow pepper
- 1 fist spinach
- 1 tomato
- 1 board of directors goat cheese
- Olive oil

Steps

1) Chop all the vegetables into small pieces
2) Beat the eggs and add the splash of milk, add pepper (you can add salt but I did not put it because it already has salty ingredients)
3) Put olive oil in the pan and add in order: onion, peppers, mushrooms, tomato and spinach
4) Add the beaten eggs covering the entire pan and cover, cook over low heat
5) Halfway through cooking add the olives, capers and goat cheese, cover and finish cooking
6) Serve with a little balsamic oil

Mediterranean shrimp

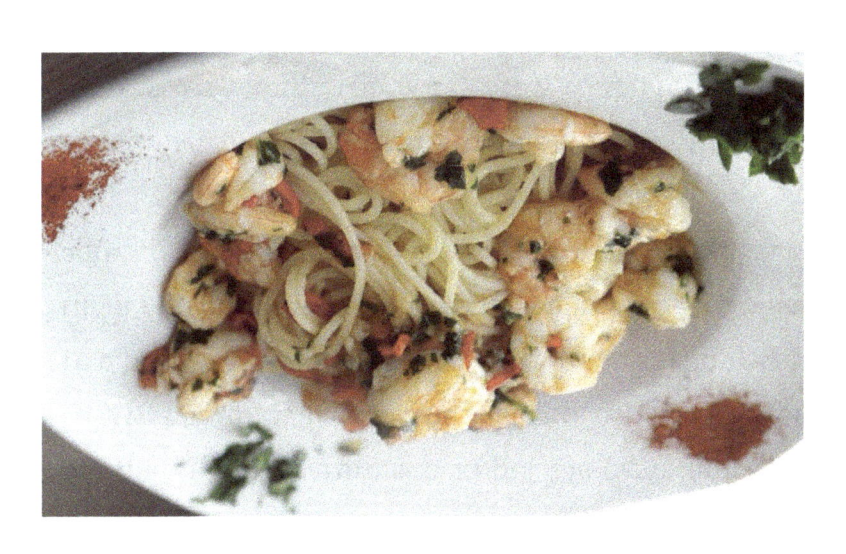

Time: 30- 40 minutes

Servings: 2

Ingredients

- 100 g spaghetti N° 5
- 20 raw medium shrimp
- 20 gr Margarine
- Fine herbs
- Maggi sauce
- 7 medium mushrooms
- sour cream

Steps

1) Wash and cut the shrimp in half, cleaning them inside.
2) Slice the mushrooms (roll).

3) Heat water to the point that it boils, once it passes, put the pasta for 9 minutes, once that time is over, put the pasta at a temperature shock, put the pasta quickly in cold water, this will make the pasta not cook completely.

4) In a pan, melt the margarine and add the shrimp, sauté them and add fine herbs (1/2 tablespoon) once cooked add the mushrooms and sauté them, add Maggi sauce, 5 shaken approximately.

5) In another pan you put margarine and add the pasta, move it with tongs, (do not beat) with the tongs, move it a minute and add the sour cream, 2 tablespoons. Mix the pasta well with the cream, once done add fine herbs (1/2 tablespoon) pepper to taste and a little salt, then add the shrimp and mushrooms, stir and that's it.

6) You can accompany it with bolillo strips and a molcajete sauce.

Greek or Mediterranean Sandwich

Time: 15 minutes

Servings: 2

Ingredients

- 8 slices Box bread
- 100g goat cheese
- 1/3 cup cream / born
- 1 tooth finely minced garlic
- 1/2 cdts ground oregano
- 1/3 cup chopped black olives
- 1 canned red bell pepper, sliced
- 1 board of directors balsamic vinegar
- 2 cdts chopped parsley
- 3 cdas olive oil
- salt and pepper to taste for seasoning

Steps

1) Chop the pepper slices, season and bathe with a little oil and vinegar.
2) Mix the cheese with the cream, add the garlic and oregano, add salt and pepper to taste.
3) Add the olives and peppers to the cheese.
4) Spread the bread slices with the cheese mixture and make a sandwich.

5) Put on a baking sheet and put them at 1500 C to lightly toast.

6) To finish, spread the parsley on the sandwiches.

Mediterranean salad

Time: 50 minutes

Servings: 6

Ingredients

- 6 tomatoes peeled, seeded and chopped
- 1 cup chopped basil leaves
- 1 cup pitted olives
- 1 tablespoon crushed oregano
- 150grms. dry cheese
- 3 tablespoons olive oil
- 2 tablespoons balsamic vinegar
- C/n salt and pepper

Steps

1) Put the tomatoes cut into wedges in a bowl.
2) Rinse the olives and cut in half.
3) Cut the cheese into cubes.
4) Mix the tomatoes, olives, cheese, add the basil leaves, mix the oil with the vinegar, oregano, salt and pepper.
5) Bathe the salad, and the best way is to mix with your hands.
6) Bon Appetite.

Mediterranean pasta

Time: 50 minutes

Servings: 6

Ingredients

- 500 grms noodles
- 1 large onion, diced
- 1 green bell pepper, chopped
- 5 teeth minced garlic
- 1 cup clean and filleted mushrooms
- 1 kilogram tomatoes
- to taste romero
- 1 cup clean, disinfected and chopped parsley
- 1 cup pitted olives
- 3 tablespoons olive oil
- 1/3 cup Water
- C/n salt and pepper
- To taste Parmesan

Steps

1) In a large pot, heat the oil, add the onion, when it bursts add the garlic and pepper, mix and cook for 5 minutes.
2) Quarter the tomatoes with a little water, blend, strain and bring to the vegetables, cook for about 10 minutes, leave a thick sauce, add the rosemary, salt and pepper.

Cook for another 10 minutes and add the mushrooms and olives.

3) Cook the pasta according to the manufacturer's instructions. Let it be al dente. Drain.

4) Put the pasta in a large plate, pour the sauce and sprinkle the parsley, remove the rosemary.

5) Add Parmesan cheese.

6) Bon Appetite.

Mediterranean salad spinach

Time: 15 min

Servings: 2

Ingredients

- 10 pzas. Spinach
- 1/2pc. Purple lettuce
- 1/2pc. Romaine lettuce
- 10pzas. Jitomate cherry (miniature)
- 1/4pc. Purple Onion
- 1/2pc. Apple
- 150 gr. Feta cheese
- 1/2oz. Balsamic vinagre
- 2 pzas. Garlic cloves
- 10pzas. Green olives
- 5pzas. Black olive
- 1oz. Olive oil
- 1/2pc. Lemon (juice)
- Salt and freshly ground black pepper.

Steps

1) Break up the purple, romaine and spinach lettuce in a bowl, cut the onion into julienne strips, peel and cut the apple into julienne strips, add the cherry tomato and mix evenly. Reserve.

2) Finely chop the garlic, add the lemon juice, balsamic vinegar, olive oil and beat with a slotted spoon until creamy, correct the flavor by adding salt and freshly ground pepper.

3) Add the olives distributing them over the salad to obtain a balance of flavor and color, add the feta cheese crumbled and finally season with the Mediterranean vinaigrette.

Mediterranean style Fusilli salad

Time: 15 minutes

Servings: 4

Ingredients

- 250gr Fusilli
- 120gr black olives (preferably pitted) previously drained
- 1/2 onion
- 1 sprig basil
- to taste Olive oil, salt and pepper

Steps

1) Boil the pasta in 2lts or 1 and a half of water with just under a tablespoon of salt.
2) When ready, drain off all excess water.
3) Wash, dry and cut the cherry tomatoes in half and remove the seeds with a spoon.
4) Remove the first layer of the onion and cut most of it together with the basil leaves.
5) In a bowl of the appropriate size, stir all the ingredients.
6) Clever

Roast vegetables and Arabic bread

Time: 30 minutes

Servings: 2

Ingredients

- Mushrooms
- Pepper
- Chives
- Alfalfa germ
- Walnut
- Blueberry
- Butter
- Seasoning (Mediterranean)
- Hummus

Steps

1) Cut up all the vegetables and put them in the pan with butter.
2) Heat your arabic bread, top it with germ, walnut, cranberry and hummus.
3) Add seasoning to hummus or vegetables. As you prefer to combine the flavor. I used this on vegetables.

Shrimp enchiladas

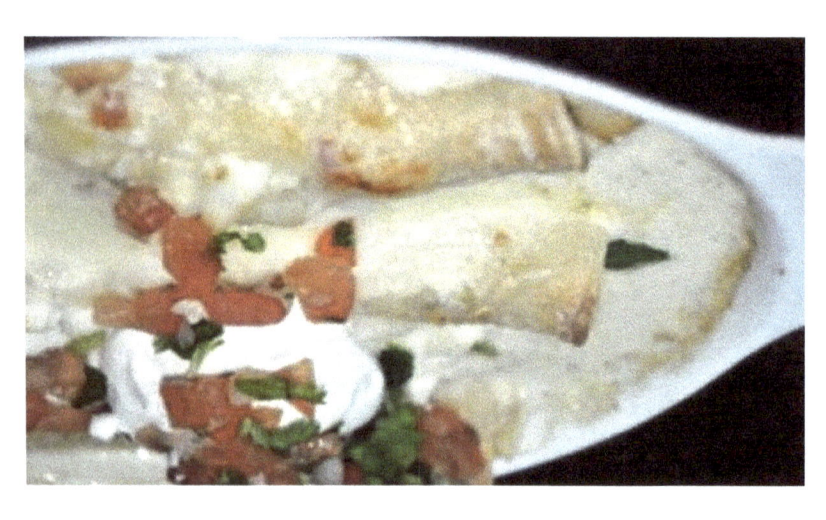

Time: 40 minutes

Servings: 1

Ingredients

- 1/4 tza onion
- 2 tomatoes
- 1 green chile
- 1/2 cdta shall
- 2 cdtas olive oil
- 10 gr Butter
- 1/2 tza leche deslactosada
- 1/3 tza tomato puree
- 80 gr delactosada cream
- 3 teeth it

- 1/3 tza cilantro
- 1/2 cdta Mediterranean mix spices
- 1/2 cdta shall
- 200 gr precooked shrimp
- 4 flour tortillas
- Cilantro for garnish

Steps

1) Finely chop the onion and chili, and dice the tomato.
2) In a skillet, heat the oil and butter. Add the onion, tomato, chili and salt. Heat for 2-3 minutes.
3) Preheat the oven to 200 ° C.
4) Mix the cream, milk, puree, garlic, coriander, spices and salt. Add the mixture and shrimp to the skillet with the vegetables. Increase the heat to a boil and then cook over medium heat for 5 minutes or until the sauce thickens.
5) Heat the tortillas. Once the shrimp sauce is done, fill the tortillas and place them in a baking dish. Cover the enchiladas with the leftover sauce.
6) Bake for 15 to 18 minutes. Serve and decorate with the coriander sprigs.
7) Tip: you can add some Manchego, Monterrey Jack or Chihuahua cheese on top of the enchiladas, just before baking.

Mediterranean salad

Time: 20 minutes

Servings: 2

Ingredients

- 1 Lemon
- to taste Shall
- 1 Green and black olives
- 1 feta Cheese tray
- 10 Black Seedless Grapes
- 1 Cucumber
- 1 Oregano
- 1 Pieces of romaine lettuce
- 10 Tomate cherry
- 1/2 pineapple

Steps

1) All the ingredients are mixed last the oregano

Chickpea salad - Mediterranean

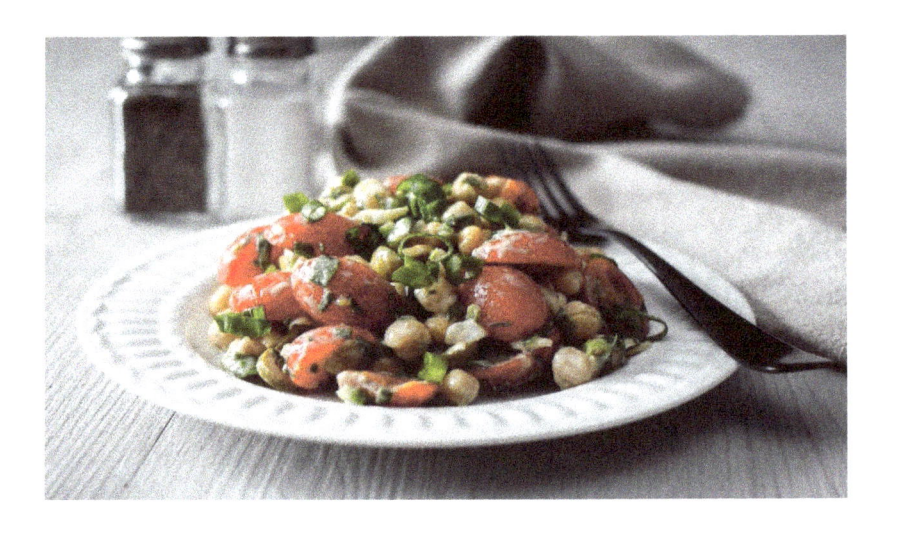

Time: 20 minutes

Servings: 2

Ingredients

- Cooked chickpeas
- Chopped tomatoes
- Chopped onion
- Chopped cucumber
- Shall
- Pepper powder

Steps

1) Add everything to a bowl and mix. Add salt just before serving so the salad isn't watery.

Mediterranean rolls

Time: 30 minutes

Servings: 4

Ingredients

- 1 sliced eggplant
- 1 board of directors cheese
- 1 1/2 cda chda de
- 5 oz cream cheese
- 1/2 roasted pepper cut into brunois
- 1cda stand or fresh basil
- for in dressing:
- 1/2 cda white vinegar, olive oil to taste a touch of pesto
- salt and pepper to taste (the ingredients are mixed and the olive oil is added in the form of a thread until emulsified)

Steps

1) The aubergine is cut into thin slices and grilled until soft.

2) Mix the cheese, the pepper and the basil, the Parmesan cheese with the mayonnaise, mix everything, wrap this mixture with the slices of aubergines and then add the dressing on top.

3) Note: the aubergines are put on a decorative toothpick to hold. If you want you can take them to the oven but it is optional.

Mediterranean beef casserole

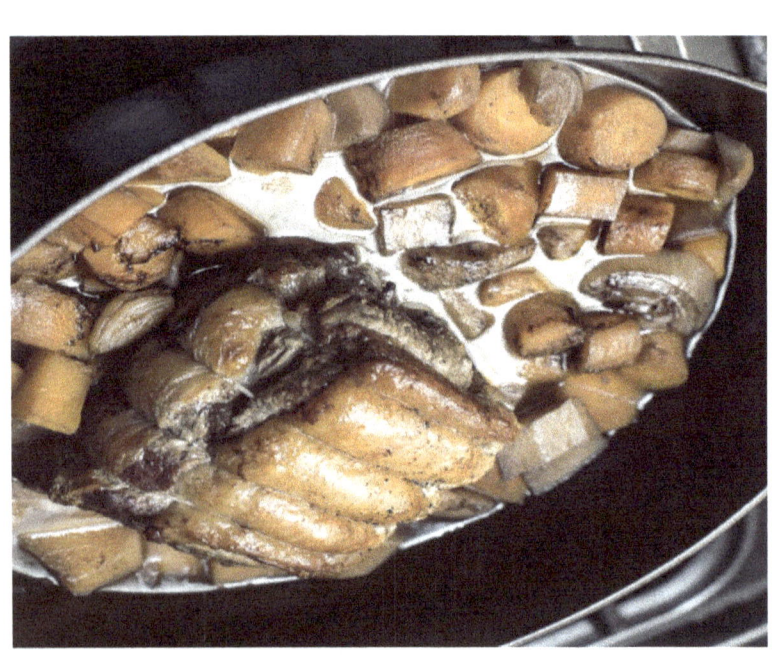

Time: 50 minutes

Servings: 6

Ingredients

- 900 gr aguayon steak (round steak moth) cut into cubes
- 2 cdas Butter
- 1 years 340 grams of tomato paste
- 2/3 cup meat broth or red wine
- 1/2 cup sliced black olives
- 2 cdas azúcar morena clara light

- 2 teeth minced garlic
- 1/4 cup red wine vinegar
- 2 leaves laurel
- 1/4 cup grapes
- 1 cdts ground cinnamon
- 1 cdts ground cloves
- 3 cups hot steamed rice

Steps

1) Preheat the oven to 375 F in a bowl, mix the steak, the melted butter, arrange in a baking dish.

2) Mix in a bowl the tomato paste, the meat broth, the vinegar, stir in the olives, the sugar, the garlic, pour over the steak. Turning it over to spread it.

3) Place bay leaves on top of meat mixture; Distribute the raisins, cinnamon, cloves on top, cover with aluminum foil.

4) Bake the casserole for 45 minutes, remove the bay leaves, discard them, arrange the cooked rice in a serving dish and spoon the meat over the rice and add salt.

Mediterranean tuna salad

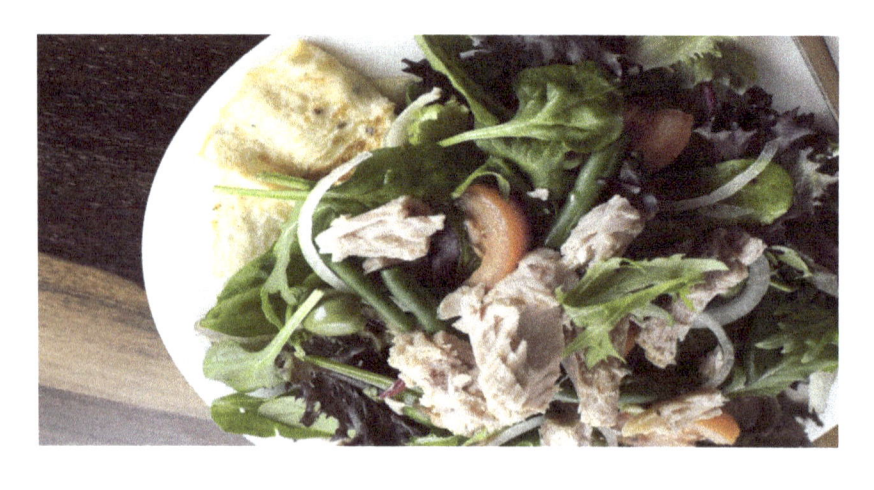

Time: 15 minutes

Servings: 2

Ingredients

- 4 cherry tomatoes, quartered
- 1 years drained tuna
- 1 sliced pickle
- 3 cdas yellow corn kernels
- 1 cdts chopped mint
- 2 cdas olive oil
- 1 board of directors lemon juice

Steps

1) Mix all the ingredients in a bowl, salt and pepper.
2) Divide them into containers and serve, accompany with crackers.

Mediterranean Screws

Time: 30 minutes

Servings: 6

Ingredients

- 1 package screw-shaped pasta
- 2 chopped sausages
- 3 poblano peppers in slices
- 1 bunch tail onions (cambray)
- 1 cup grated cheese

Steps

1) The pasta is cooked in a large saucepan in 1 1/2 liters of water with fragrant herbs and a drizzle of vegetable oil and salt.

2) In a frying pan, fry the chorizo until it is well cooked, add the filleted chambray onions and the poblano pepper slices.

3) Once the onion is seasoned, add the freshly cooked pasta, properly drained, add all the ingredients, put the grated cheese on top and cook for 5 minutes. Garnish with parsley and grated cheese.

Mediterranean chicken with 4 cheeses

Time: 15 minutes

Servings: 4

Ingredients

- 4 halves boneless, skinless small breasts
- 1 years diced tomatoes
- 1/2 cup chopped black olives
- 1 board of directors grated lemon peel
- 1 cup cinco quesos finely, shedded, italian, five, cheese y blend
- In some supermarkets they all come in a bag

Steps

1) The breasts are fried in little oil for 7 minutes on each side, or until cooked.
2) Add diced tomatoes, grated lemon peel and cook for 5 minutes.
3) This mixture is added to the chicken and it is brought to the fire for 2 minutes until everything has been well mixed, and the cheeses are added to the last.
4) It is served with screw paste and is also drizzled with tomato sauce.

Grape salad

Time: 20 minutes

Servings: 3

Ingredients

- 30 grapes
- Green olives
- Mediterranean cheese
- 1 Feta cheese
- 1 Red onion
- 1 Cucumber
- 1 Lettuce mesclum
- 1/2 Oregano in envelope
- 3 lemons
- 3 tablespoons extra virgin olive oil
- 3 tablespoons wine vinegar
- 1 pinch salt and pepper
- 30 tomatoes cherry

Steps

1) Cut and mix all the ingredients last add the oregano

Slow Baked Beef

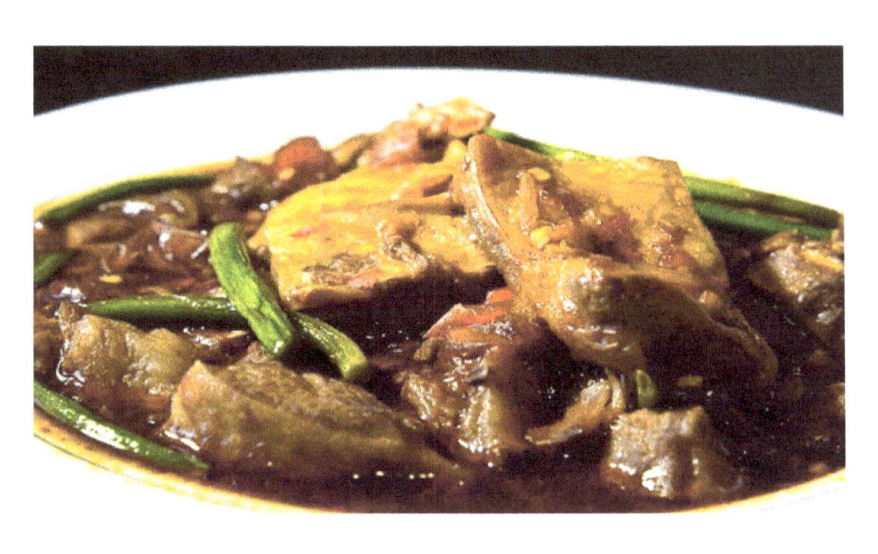

Time: 70 minutes

Servings: 5

Ingredients

- lbs beef brisket
- to taste Mediterranean sal
- 5 teeth it
- 1 board of directors ground onion
- 1 jet vinegar
- 1 board of directors salsa worcestershire
- 1 cdita ground cumin
- 1 jet red table wine
- 1 board of directors mustard
- 1 board of directors Oyster sauce

Steps

1) Clean the meat and cut it into pieces to taste.
2) Then season and bake at 375F for 30 minutes, flip. Bake an additional 30 minutes.
3) If your family likes tender meat, depending on the thickness, you may need to transfer it to the speed cooker. Cook 7 minutes at high temperature.
4) Serve with boiled green bananas or rice.

Baked Chicken in its Juice

Time: 70 minutes

Servings: 4

Ingredients

- 8 chicken thighs
- 1 board of directors ground dried garlic
- 1 board of directors ground dried onion
- 1 board of directors ground celery seed
- 1 board of directors mediterranean oil
- Complete ground seasoning
- 1 board of directors seasoned salt
- Spray oil
- Vinegar water

Steps

1) Rinse the pieces in cold water, drain and soak in vinegar water for 10 minutes.

2) In a tray with a wire rack preferably, so that the fat drips off, suitable for the oven, spray the bottom with the cooking spray.

3) Season, making sure you cover the chicken well and place the pieces. Then bake at 375°F for 30 minutes. Flip and bake 20-25 minutes or until cooked through. Serve immediately, accompanied by boiled vegetables.

Beef Meatballs in Vegetable Bath

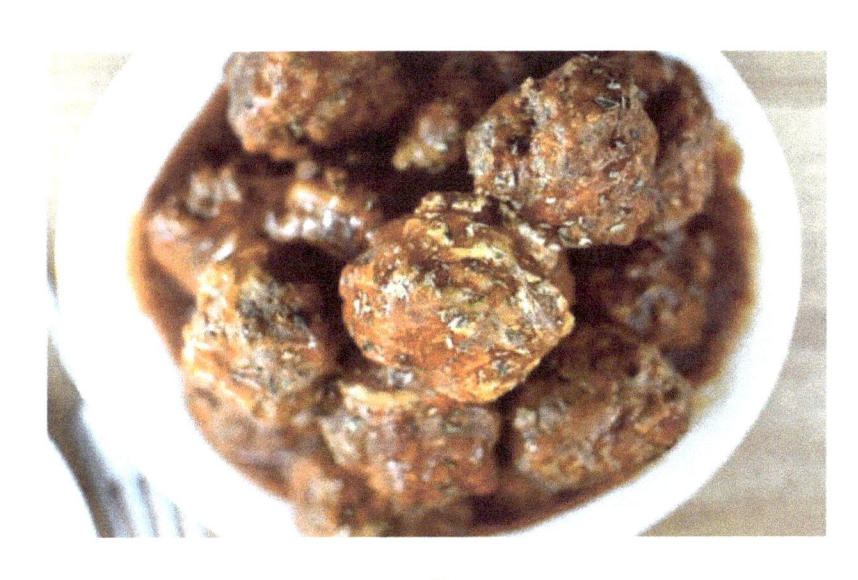

Time: 70 minutes

Servings: 6

Ingredients

- 1/2 Bell pepper
- 1/2 stem celery
- 3 teeth natural garlic
- 3 teeth roasted garlic
- Chicken broth to blend the seasonings
- 4 ripe bululu tomatoes
- 1 board of directors Mediterranean oil (canola-grapeseed-extra virgin olive) to fry the seasoning

- 14 large beef meatballs (baseball size)
- 16 oz of diced tomatoes with their juice
- 1 pinch ground turmeric
- 1 pinch ground cumin
- 1 cdita ground onion
- 16 ounces chickpeas cooked and drained
- Chicken broth as required.
- 1 cup carrots in thick wheels
- 6 chunks potatoes the size of 1 baseball
- 1 cup butternut squash peeled and in pieces

Steps

1) Process the seasoning (the first 6 ingredients) and the tomatoes, in the blender, covering with liquid chicken broth.
2) In the pot that you will prepare the broth, pour the oil and fry the liquefied seasoning.
3) Uniting, fry for 1 minute. Add the meatballs, use pre-cooked and frozen. This speeds up the preparation process. Continue sautéing and joining.
4) Then add the carrot, chicken broth (I used homemade broth) but you can use whatever you like. Add water to get the desired consistency. Squash into pieces. Potatoes in large chunks. The tomato can and the drained chickpeas.

5) Add the turmeric and cumin, after tasting.

6) Lower heat and cook until the vegetables are tender.

7) When you turn off the heat, add a sprig of thyme and oregano, preferably natural. Cover and let stand for 10 minutes before serving.

8) It depends on the meat and personal taste, the fat is removed using a fat separator or letting it cool because the fat floats on top and thus you remove it.

9) Accompany with white rice or bread.

Rice with Smoked Sausages and Beer

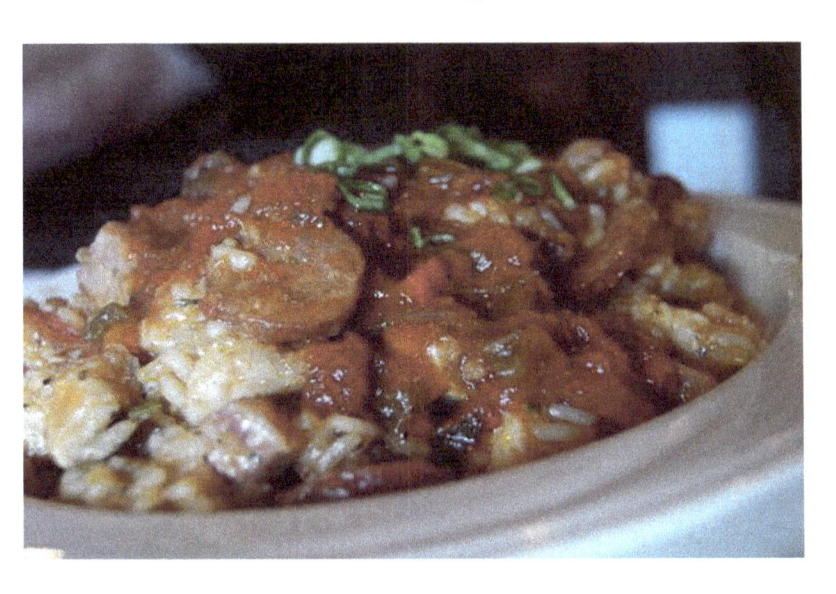

Time: 30 minutes

Servings: 4

Ingredients

- 14 oz smoked beef sausage
- 3 1/2 cups raw rice
- 1/2 onion in small cubes
- 1/2 bell pepper in small cubes
- 1 board of directors crushed garlic
- 1 bucket chicken soup
- 1/4 cup ketchup
- water to prepare the rice

- 1 board of directors Mediterranean oil (olive-canola-grapeseed)

Steps

1) You add the oil to the pot you use, I personally prefer the speed cooker for its convenience. Heat over medium heat, add the onion, bell pepper and garlic, sauté, mixing well.

2) add the sausages, continue sautéing until they have browned, the tomato sauce, continue to join.

3) Drizzle the stream of beer and continue mixing while sautéing. And you let the alcohol evaporate

4) the rice, combine well and sauté for approximately 1 minute.

5) add enough water to prepare the rice, this will depend on the pot you are using.

6) taste of salt and cook like normal rice.

Red beef tail

Time: 50 minutes

Servings: 4

Ingredients

- 4 lbs Clean beef tail
- 2 Large onions
- 1 Aji morron
- Flour for dusting the meat
- 3 teeth it
- 3/4 cup Red wine
- Salt taste salt
- 1 pinch Ground paprika
- 4 Tomatoes or equivalent tomato sauce
- to taste Parsley
- 1/4 cdita Dried ground turmeric
- to taste Freshly ground pepper
- Natural water as needed
- 1/2 cdita Ground dried oregano
- 2 cdas Mediterranean oil (olive-grapeseed-canola)

Steps

1) Rinse the tail in vinegar water. dry well. Brush the tail with salt and flour.

2) You heat the oil in the pot. Sauté the meat in the pan in a few portions until golden, while turning it.

3) Onion, garlic, pasta or tomatoes, bell pepper, paprika, oregano, parsley, turmeric, you process it into a sauce. You add the water as required.

4) Cover the bottom of the pot with the sauce, add the tail. Pour the excess sauce over the meat.

5) You rectify the salt, add the wine, mix well and close. In the pressure cooker you give it 30 minutes at high temperature. In a regular pot 1 1/2 hours. Try pricking with a fork, if it is soft, it is ready to enjoy, accompanied by a white rice, preferably.

Oven fried chicken thigh

Time: 70 minutes

Servings: 4

Ingredients

- 10 chicken thighs
- mustard to cover the thighs
- 1 jet rice vinegar for seasoning
- 1 jet apple cider vinegar to wash the bird
- to taste garlic powder
- to taste onion powder
- to taste full seasoning without powdered salt
- to taste ground salt
- 2 cups wheat flour
- Ground dried rosemary
- ground dried parsley
- 2 beaten eggs
- peanut oil
- Mediterranean oil (olive-canola-grape seed) or olive oil, for seasoning

Steps

1) Clean and rinse in apple cider vinegar water for a few minutes. Drain or pat dry with a paper towel.

2) Season with the ingredients except the parsley, rosemary, peanut oil, flour and eggs. Keep covered for 15 minutes so that it takes the seasoning.

3) Piece by piece go through the beaten egg, then through the flour that you will have prepared with the parsley and rosemary and through the egg mixture, shake off excess.

4) Place on an oven-safe tray that you will have previously greased. Drizzle peanut oil on the chicken after placing it on the tray. We bake at a temperature of 375F for 30 minutes and then turn and rise to 380F for 15-20 minutes or until both sides are golden brown and cooked on the inside.

Moro Red Beans with Salami Genoa

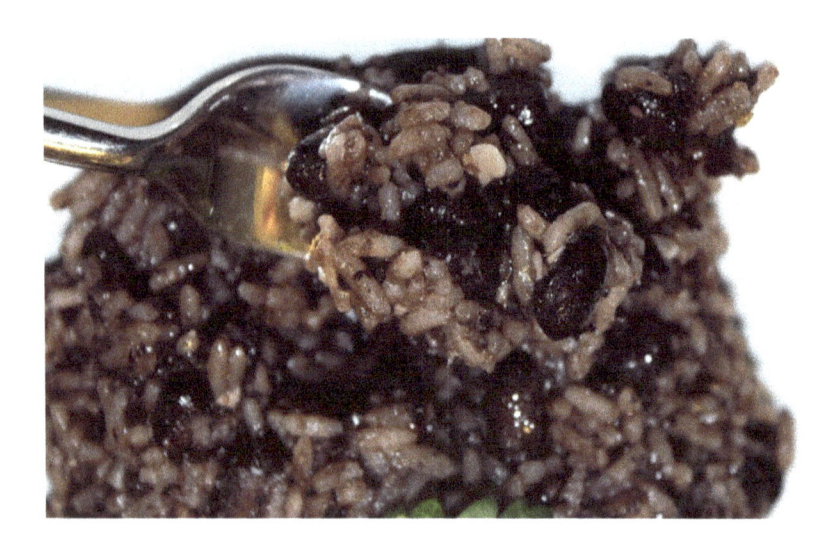

Time: 20 minutes

Servings: 4

Ingredients

- 3 cups raw rice
- 6 slices Salami Genoa
- 1 tablet chicken soup
- 2 each pico de gallo (onion-tomatoes-coriander-lemon juice)
- Mediterranean blend oil
- 1/2 cup ketchup
- 4 cups natural water
- 2 cupsRed beans boiled but firm. Or a rinsed can of beans

Steps

1) In a tablespoon of Mediterranean oil (mixture of - grapeseed-extra virgin olive- canola), sauté the pico de gallo over medium heat, for a minute, then add the tomato sauce while continuing to sauté. Continuing with the beans, keep moving.

2) Rinse the rice and add to the pot, you are sautéing while you turn.

3) Heat the water and add the chicken broth tablet, dissolve.

4) When you have sautéed the rice and beans, for about 2 minutes, add the water to completely cover the mixture and cook like ordinary rice.

5) I made it in a quick cooker, it also makes perfect on the stovetop.

6) Add a drizzle of olive oil when serving.

Dominican style coconut fish

Time: 30 minutes

Servings: 4

Ingredients:

- 8 steaks White fish
- 1 Large onion julienned or diced
- 1 Large red bell pepper, julienned
- 1 board of directors Ground garlic and two minced garlic cloves
- 1 sprig Fresh rosemary or 1 teaspoon dried
- 1 cdita Ground turmeric or annatto
- 2 cda Mediterranean oil (olive-canola-seed grapes) or equivalent
- 1 board of directors Coriander, if dry only 1 / 2cdita
- 1 cup Coconut milk to taste
- 1 cdita chicken broth paste or equivalent
- to taste Shall

Steps

1) Rinse the fish with cold water. Pat dry with a paper towel. Cut into medium pieces. Unes salt, garlic powder, turmeric or annatto. You season the fish with that mixture.

2) In a frying pan, heat the oil and place the garlic, onion and bell pepper cut into julienne strips. Sauté until the onion is shiny. Add the chicken broth paste or full seasoning

3) Add the fish and turn several times, joining with the onion and peppers. You add the coconut milk, lower the heat and cook until the milk is half consumed.

4) Salt tests and add chopped cilantro. Serve alongside rice.

Mediterranean salad

Time: 15 min

Servings: 2

Ingredients

- 150 grs cooked green beans
- 1/2 palta
- 4 olives
- 1/4 purple Onion
- 1 slice feta cheese
- Juice of 1 lemon
- Salt, oil and pepper

Steps

1) Cook the beans, I used frozen because around here in Punta Arenas it is difficult to get fresh, but if you have fresh it is better. Leave al dente, cool and arrange in a salad bowl. Chop the other ingredients to taste. Season with salt, pepper, lemon and olive oil and serve. It is very delicious, the sheep's feta cheese gives it the maximum touch.

Mediterranean Fish Casserole

Time: 40 minutes

Servings: 6

Ingredients

- 1 kg dogfish
- 1 big Onion
- 1 bell pepper
- 4 medium potatoes
- 1 carrot
- Seasonings Garlic, oregano etc
- 1/4 cup flour
- 2 tomatoes
- 1 cup ketchup
- 1 cup wine

Steps

1) Chop the onion, bell pepper, carrot and fry in a saucepan over low heat.
2) We add the chopped tomato, the seasonings and the wine.
3) Then the potatoes and the tomato sauce. When they are almost cooked we incorporate the fish posts, before we pass them through flour so that they do not fall apart
4) We leave 10 more minutes and serve in casseroles

5) Deli remains! Enjoy

Mediterranean spoons

Time: 30 minutes

Servings: 4

Ingredients

- leaves basil
- tomates cherry
- boconccinos or mozzarella

Steps

1) Wash, dry, put basil leaves at the base of the spoon
2) Top a boconccino or a piece of mozzarella, cover with another basil leaf
3) Cut the cherry tomato lengthwise, place it on the cheese, finish with a basil leaf - click with a toothpick to join
4) It begins and ends with a basil leaf and in the middle of the ingredients - season and sprinkle with just a few drops of olive
5) They lean on the spoons but take it, grab the toothpick and eat it in one bite - the toothpick is put back on the spoon

Mediterranean salad in low cholesterol

Time: 30 minutes

Servings: 3

Ingredients

- 1 pair of leaves (large) kale in thin strips
- 4 sheets red lettuce in rustic pieces
- 8 sheets arugula, tender in rustic chunks
- 8-12 sliced black olives
- 200 grams fresh mushrooms filleted
- 1 sweet Catalan chili pepper, peeled, seeded and cut into strips f
- 3 generous tablespoons Olive oil
- Get out what is necessary
- Garlic 2 whole cloves
- Fresh herbs thyme, oregano, and parsley, finely chopped
- About 18 sheets basil, some (9 whole, others finely chopped)
- 1 splash Alcohol vinegar
- 2 tablespoons Soy sauce
- 1 tsp sugar girl
- 4 thin fetas Parmesan
- 1 tablespoon peeled and sliced almonds

- 1 pinch Freshly ground black pepper
- 1 slice manteca

Steps

1) We wash, peel and cut the vegetables as mentioned above. For the dressing we put in a bowl: olives, the finely chopped herbs, the soy sauce, olive oil / season, add the vinegar and emulsify well. Meanwhile we toast the sliced almonds. Reserve

2) Having thoroughly washed the arugula, lettuce, kale (in thin strips) and about 9 basil leaves, we cut them into rustic pieces (by hand) we put them in a salad bowl to which the raw garlic previously passed to take flavor. We add the four slices of Parmesan cheese. We booked.

3) In a pan with olive oil and a bit of butter, we wait for it to warm ... we add the Catalan chili pepper, the two whole cloves of garlic, brown for about 4 minutes, then add the mushrooms.

4) The mushrooms are very clean, they are not washed, filleted ... we mix them with the sweet pepper and leave for about 5 minutes, add the finely chopped herbs, basil, oregano, thyme and parsley, season and mix well. We withdraw ... and RESERVE UNTIL THEY COOL IN A BOLS.When the mushrooms are cold we add to the

salad bowl that has the leaves and the Parmesan cheese, add the dressing and mix carefully, not much.

5) Add the toasted and sliced almonds, serve

Mediterranean orzo pasta salad

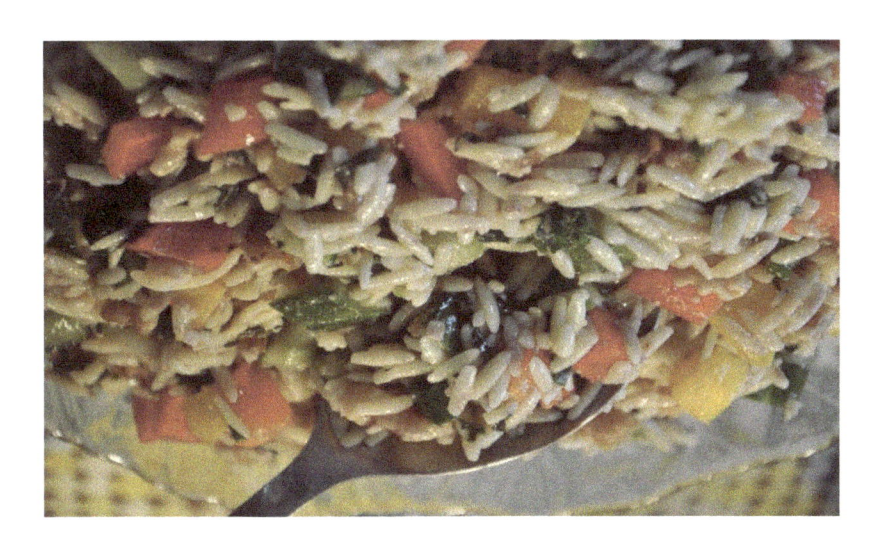

Time: 20 min

Servings: 3

Ingredients

- Tomates cherry
- Green pepper
- Tender garlic
- Cucumber
- Parsley
- Dill
- Kalamata olives
- Capers (optional)
- Barley pasta

- Olive oil, salt, pepper, lemon juice and rallasira, garlic
- feta Cheese

Steps

1) We cut some cherry tomatoes in half and a very chopped green pepper.
2) Photo of step 1 of the recipe Mediterranean orzo pasta salad
3) We also add a couple of garlic cloves.
4) A handful of finely chopped parsley.
5) And also dill, removing the stems that are thicker.
6) We add half a cucumber.
7) And the previously cooked orzo pasta that we had allowed to cool a bit.
8) We stir everything well and add the salad dressing that we have prepared.
9) We have done it with a good jet of olive oil, lemon juice and zest, finely minced garlic cloves, salt and pepper.
10) We add some black olives and feta cheese.
11) And here we have the result, an orzo salad with Mediterranean flavors.

Mediterranean toast with seeds

Time: 20 min

Servings: 3

Ingredients

- 2 slices poppy seed bread
- 1 ripe Mancate avocado
- espinacas baby
- 8-10 pitted black olives
- 1 tablespoon seeds (sunflower, sesame, flax, pumpkin, poppy)
- salt grinder and 5 peppers
- Extra virgin olive

Steps

1) Wash and dry the spinach leaves well. Cut the avocado into slices and the black olives.
2) Toast the bread smeared with a drop of oil and serve with the spinach, avocado, olives, seeds and a drizzle of oil on top. Season to taste.

Main course Mediterranean salad

Time: 20 minutes

Servings: 3

Ingredients

- 1 Romaine lettuce
- 1 bowl of grated beet
- 1 bean sprouts bowl
- 1 bowl of grated carrot
- 1 red or purple onion
- 1 bowl of black olives
- 1 bowl of green olives
- 1 lamb's lettuce bowl
- 3 packages surimi sticks
- 3 tuna slices in olive oil
- 3 eggs
- Extra virgin olive oil
- to taste Salt, pepper and vinegar

Steps

1) We prepare the ingredients, put the eggs to cook, cut the lettuce and put it in water with a splash of vinegar to preserve its fresh flavor, cut the onion into julienne strips.

2) Cut the crab surimi, put the lettuce in the centrifuge, spin the lettuce and put it in a bowl

3) And we are adding ingredients the onion the lamb's lettuce the surimi the bean sprouts the grated beet the carrot the red and green olives

4) We move it well, put it in individual bowls, add the tuna, the quartered eggs and some strips of roasted peppers and enjoy a complete salad.

Mediterranean salad with Cheese

Time: 10 minutes

Servings: 2

Ingredients

- 1 Lettuce
- 1 or 2 coat
- 1 slice cheese
- 1 cup Valencian olives
- 1/2 Yellow bell
- 10 radish
- Fennel, tarragon
- pink salt
- olive oil
- lemon juice

Steps

1) Wash and chop the ingredients to taste and add seasonings and herbs to taste.
2) Garnish with yellow bell pepper and radish.

Mediterranean pasta tomatoes

Time: 30 minutes

Servings: 5

Ingredients

- 1 package spaghetti (or whatever pasta you want)
- 10 cherry tomatoes (the 2 large tomatoes)
- satisfaced Basil leaves
- satisfaced condiments
- 1 tray fresh portobellos

Steps

1) Let's cut the tomatoes and portobellos into cubes in half (or as you prefer)
2) We take a large pot and with butter (or oil) we sauté the portobellos.
3) Once ready, add plenty of water and wait for it to boil.
4) Add the pasta and wait until they are ready.
5) Now it's time to add the tomatoes, and the basil.
6) We wait for the water to be finished, season to taste and voila!

Murcian Mediterranean Pizza

Time: 15 minutes

Servings: 4

Ingredients:

- 1 Homemade pizza dough
- 2 cans tuna
- 1/2 Red pepper
- 1/2 green pepper
- 1/2 yellow pepper
- Sausage turkey breast
- 1 onion
- 100 gr mushroom
- Sliced cheese
- 1 tarrina bacon cut into strips

Steps

1) Make the dough and let it rest for 20 minutes
2) It stretches and goes to the llanda. The oven is preheated up and down to the top. Then it goes down to 180 degrees
3) I stir-fry green, red, yellow peppers, onions. Then the mushroom. I leave it on absorbent paper. (I pass it on for the iron, since they leave water and if not, the dough would cost to make or it would come out soft)

4) Tomato oregano is added

5) All the ingredients are added. Sausage turkey breast, tuna, bacon, red, green, yellow pepper, mushroom, green olive cheese and baked. Approx 180 grad 30 to 40 minutes

6) And made mmmm delicious

Mediterranean chickpea and pasta salad

Time: 15 minutes

Servings: 4

Ingredients:

- 400 gr cooked chickpeas
- 150 gr vegetable bow ties
- black olives
- corn cobs
- dried tomato in oil
- canons
- Extra virgin olive oil DO Montes de Toledo
- lemon juice
- fresh parsley
- Sea Salt with Chimichurri from Salinas de Janubio
- fresh red chilli

Steps

1) Drain and wash the chickpeas well without being canned. If not, cook in white (water + salt + bay leaf). Cook the pasta in boiling water and slightly salted according to the manufacturer's recommendation.

2) Mix all the ingredients and reserve. In a jar with a lid, put the oil, lemon juice, chopped parsley, chopped chilli

and the salt with chimichurri, close and shake for a few seconds. Drizzle the salad with the dressing.

Baked Mediterranean Skimmed

Time: 70 minutes

Servings: 2

Ingredients

- 2 large eggplants
- 1 large paprika
- 1 big Onion
- 1 big tomato
- Salt and olive oil
- Vinaigrette
- 1 tsp balsamic vinegar
- 1 pinch shall
- to taste Oregano
- Pepper
- 1 tsp olive oil
- 1 tablespoon honey

Steps

1) Wash the vegetables and make small cuts on the skin (reserve the tomato) sprinkle salt and olive oil, put in the oven for 50 minutes at 180 degrees, turning, after 50 minutes put the tomatoes for 20 more minutes with the vegetables. Turn off and let it rest.

2) Drain the liquids released by the vegetables into a container and reserve, remove the skin from the vegetables and cut them into strips or julienne strips and plate.

3) For the vinaigrette we take the liquids of the vegetables, add a pinch of salt, balsamic vinegar, honey, pepper, oregano and stir, add the olive oil and bathe our roasted vegetables, you will not stop eating, We accompany it with white rice and grilled breast.

Mediterranean roast chicken chickpea salad

Time: 30 minutes

Servings: 3

Ingredients

- 1 bote cooked chickpeas
- Lemon juice
- 1 ripe tomato
- 1/2 small onion or chive
- Cilantro
- 100 gr feta cheese
- Canned tuna or in my case some leftover roast chicken
- Salt, pepper and dried oregano
- aove
- Balsamic vinegar

Steps

1) We drain the chickpeas in a colander and wash well so that no remains of the canning liquid remain, then we dehydrate them in a frying pan without oil and without anything, when we see that there are remaining retinues (no more than 5-6 min) we add some drops of squeezed lemon

2) Once we have the chickpeas ready, we transfer them to a bowl or source, and while they are tempering, we cut a tomato and small cubes, the same chives and a handful of fresh coriander too, all well chopped

3) It is time to add the canned tuna, previously drained or in my case, some remains of roast chicken that I had in the freezer, we crumble it well and add to the previous mixture

4) For the dressing, season with salt, pepper and oregano to taste, extra virgin olive oil and balsamic vinegar. When we serve it on the plate, we will add the crumbled feta cheese and we will only have to enjoy this platazo

Mediterranean salad with tomatoes

Time: 15 minutes

Servings: 2-3

Ingredients

- 2 salad florets
- Cherry tomatoes of assorted colors
- 1 latita olives stuffed with bell pepper
- 1/2 purple Onion
- 1 bote alcachofas baby
- Sultanas raisins
- 1 years mackerel in oil
- Aove
- Shall
- Lemon juice

Steps

1) Wash and cut the florets, put them in a bowl and add the other ingredients, the tomatoes, the onion, the olives, the artichokes, and the raisins.
2) Dress with the oil, salt and lemon, mix and add the pieces of mackerel and enjoy it because it is delicious.

Mediterranean Bruschetta

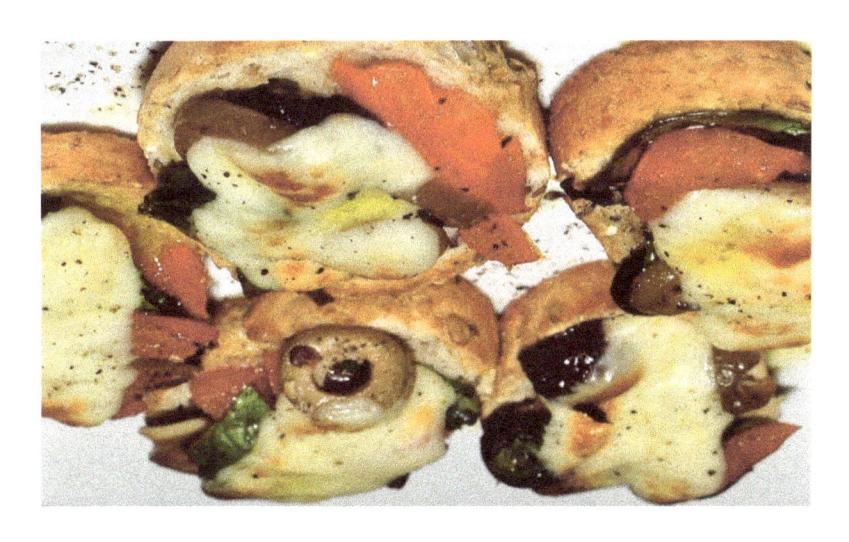

Time: 20 minutes

Servings: 2

Ingredients

- 4 slices table bread
- Black olives (10)
- 6 fetted mushrooms
- Provencal at ease
- 4 slices Mozzarella cheese (I used pulpet)
- 1 board of directors grated cheese

Steps

1) First cut the bread slices, spread them with olive oil and a little spice on top. It can be oregano. I used salt with

herbs. It is very important not to toast the bread, remove it as soon as the edges are crisp.

2) Sauté the mushrooms with the olive in a little olive oil and Provençal to taste.

3) On the bread, put the slice of mozzarella, a little black pepper from above if you wish, then the sautéed, and to finish, put the grated cheese.

CONCLUSION

The Mediterranean diet references some characteristic eating habits; it is also a cultural model that involves the way foods are selected, produced, processed, and distributed. The Mediterranean dietary pattern is presented as a cultural model and a healthy and environmentally friendly model. UNESCO recognition of the Mediterranean diet as an Intangible Cultural Heritage of Humanity represents strong visibility and acceptance of the Mediterranean diet worldwide. This, along with better and more scientific evidence relating its benefits and effects on longevity, quality of life, and disease prevention, has taken this dietary pattern to a historical moment without precedent. This is a positive situation that could empower the Mediterranean diet around the world, thereby enhancing global health indicators and decreasing environmental impact by production and transportation of food resources. To this end, the Mediterranean diet should be seen for what it is: an extremely and incomparable healthy, affordable and environmentally sustainable food model, as well as an ancient cultural heritage that confers identity and belonging. From the heart to the earth through the road of culture, the Mediterranean diet is a cultural heritage that looks to the future.

CPSIA information can be obtained
at www.ICGtesting.com
Printed in the USA
BVHW091529270521
608293BV00004B/999